# Nature's Remedy for Hypothyroidism

## *Curing Thyroid Problems Safely and Effectively Without Hurting Your Pocket*

# Disclaimer and Terms of Use

Effort has been made to ensure that the information in this book is accurate and complete, however, the author and the publisher do not warrant the accuracy of the information, text and graphics contained within the book due to the rapidly changing nature of science, research, known and unknown facts and internet. The Author and the publisher do not hold any responsibility for errors, omissions or contrary interpretation of the subject matter herein. This book is presented solely for motivational and informational purposes only.

# Contents

# Introduction

With the fast paced nature of most societies, people can't afford to get sick; a good citizen is a productive citizen. Because of this ideology that has been widely accepted in most cultures, people search for quick fixes when their body breaks down.

Western medicine has been the saving grace of people who just can't miss a single day of work. If you have high blood pressure, take a pill. If you have cancer, go through chemotherapy. Western medicine is a powerful tool in getting rid of symptoms of disease fast. Having started only in the 19th century, western medicine made quite an impressive feat.

While Western Medicine has been hailed for being very potent, it's not without its kinks. For example, when a patient is sick he has to tell the doctor what kind of pain he feels and where he feels it. That may be acceptable if everybody had the same threshold of pain and could properly describe his disease. In most cases though, doctors prescribe based on what the patient says and in a lot of cases, the prescription only gets rid of the symptoms and not the actual cause of the disease.

The body is an amazing interconnection of systems. The interconnection is so complex that it can be particularly difficult to diagnose and repair your body when it breaks down. When the body is not functioning properly, it sends out a lot of signals that can be quite difficult to interpret. A certain disease may cause symptoms of some other disease to manifest. Since a lot of medicines usually just get rid of symptoms, feeling better won't necessarily mean that you really are better.

People get various types of discomfort as they grow older. Lack of energy, lower sex drive, and moodiness are just a few of the inconveniences accepted to happen when you're past your prime. That's not all though; hypertension is one of the most common ailments that afflict more than 50% of the American population aged over 60. Most of these people are subjected to a lifetime of expensive medication, and oftentimes these medications have plenty of adverse side effects.

The thyroid gland is a very small yet very important part of the body. Problems with this gland could cause congestion in the blood vessels, slow healing of wounds, and more. Its role is so important that it can cause your whole body to break down if it malfunctions. In fact, a lot of the problems encountered by older people could come from the thyroid gland not doing its job properly.

In this book, you'll discover what the thyroid gland does and how it works with the rest of the body. You'll also learn about various diseases, their surprising correlation with a low thyroid function and how to heal and protect yourself from thyroid problems. To wrap it up, you'll also learn how to shield yourself from various health myths about the thyroid gland and how to be more vigilant in selecting cures and remedies. Various unfounded myths and profit-oriented products can cloud the path to great health. This book aims to bring nature back to the equation. It's time to bring the power of healing back to the body.

# Chapter 1: The Thyroid Gland

A lot of people have heard of the word "thyroid" but oftentimes, they don't really know what it does or what its uses are... until it breaks down, that is. The thyroid gland is a small gland shaped like a bowtie or a butterfly. It's wrapped around the windpipe just below the Adam's apple producing several hormones, the most notable ones being triiodothyronine (T3) and thyroxine (T4).

**Thyroid Gland and Thyroid Hormones: an Indepth Discussion**

It's important to understand at a cellular level how thyroid hormones are produced and how the thyroid gland makes them. When you understand this, you'll be able to make smarter decisions for better health. You'll also be able to protect yourself from various myths.

A lot of the metabolic processes in your body are regulated by the thyroid hormones triidothyronine (T3) and thyroxine (T4) that are produced by the thyroid gland. If you zoom in your throat, you'd be able to see the thyroid gland situated just below the larynx and above the trachea connecting to the lungs. Zooming in further, you'd find a structure that looks sort of like a bunch of pearl necklaces placed beside each other. The "pearls" are what you'd call the follicle cells and the space enclosed by these "pearls" is called a colloid. These follicle cells produce the T3 and T4 that increase metabolic rate among a few other things.

**What stimulates the production of these two hormones?**

The thyroid gland doesn't produce the hormones all on its own – it gets instructions from another unit. The endocrine system manages hormone production in the body. Most likely you've heard of the term "hormone" a lot of times especially during your teens. An imbalance of hormones can cause instantaneous energy loss and even mood swings, which is why the hypothalamus is in charge of stimulating the glands. It has two lobes underneath it called the anterior pituitary gland and the inferior pituitary gland.

The hypothalamus sends out thyroid-releasing hormones (TRH) to tell the anterior pituitary gland to send out thyroid-stimulating hormones (TSH). TSHs then tell the thyroid gland to produce the thyroid hormones T3 and T4.

The thyroid gland will just do as it's told unless it's malfunctioning. The hypothalamus is the one that releases less TRH when T3 and T4 are too many.

**How are Thyroid Hormones Synthesized?**

If we zoom into a particular part of the "pearl necklace" structure, we'd be able to see how thyroid hormones are synthesized. Imagine a couple of threads forming circles around the pearl necklace. Those are the blood vessels. Inside them there are plenty of molecules such as iodide, sodium, and potassium.

Inside the "pearls", we have a coral-like structure called the endoplasmic reticulum. It's in charge of packing stuff with the help of the Golgi apparatus. It transports thyroglobulin, a bracelet-like chain of carbons consisting of tyrosine molecules, to the center of the "pearl necklace", or the colloid.

Let's go back to the thread that circles the pearl necklace, or the blood vessels. We need iodide to synthesize thyroid hormones. Since the iodides are in the blood vessels, they need a vehicle to take them from the "thread" (blood vessels) to the "pearl" (follicular cells). This vehicle is called a sodium and iodide symporter. This vehicle transports both the sodium and iodide to the follicular cells. Now that iodide is inside the "pearl", the iodide then needs to be transported to the center of the pearl necklace (colloid) because the actual creation of thyroid hormones happens there.

The symporter can only bring sodium and iodide to the "pearl", but it can't go any further than that. Another vehicle called pendrin takes the job of transporting the iodide to the colloid while getting chlorine in exchange. Now that the iodide is in the colloid, a special enzyme called peroxidase converts iodide to iodine.

Remember the bracelet-like chain called thyroglobulin? Iodine will bind to the rings attached to it. One iodine molecule attached to one tyrosine ring is called MIT (Monoiodotyrosine), and two iodine molecules attached to one tyrosine ring is called DIT (Diiodotyrosine). Two DITs or an MIT and a DIT can form bonds with each other, therefore effectively making two tyrosine rings stick to each other. Triidothyronine (T3) is made from one MIT and one DIT bound together, which have three iodine molecules. Thyroxine is made from two DITs bound together, which have four iodine molecules.

We're not yet done! – They're still connected to the thyroglobulin. They'll be packed up into the "pearl" first. Then the tyrosine molecules will be released, causing the T3 and T4 to separate, and other factors are also taken care of so that the process could start again.

**How do the thyroid hormones know where to go?**

T3 and T4 don't know how to travel alone, so they have to attach themselves to special proteins called thyroid-binding proteins. These proteins are present in the blood vessels and are therefore able to go anywhere around the body, bringing the thyroid hormones to various cells and tissues.

There are more T4 secreted by the "pearls" than T3. Approximately 93% of the thyroid hormones created are T4s, leaving a miniscule 7% for T3s. However, T3 is ten times more active than T4. Only T3 can produce the energy your body needs, so when they arrive at their target cells or tissues, T4 is converted to T3 whereas T3 remains the same.

In order to convert T4 to T3, an enzyme called deiodinase removes one iodine atom from T4, effectively converting it to T3. This happens in a lot of places in the body especially your gastrointestinal system and your liver, which is why you need to take care of all the parts of your body in order to stay healthy.

T3 and T4 enter the nucleus of their target cells. Inside it, there are two receptors for initiating transcription for thyroid hormone responses, namely the thyroid hormone receptor and the retinoid x receptor. T3 and T4 will bind to the thyroid hormone receptor, effectively promoting the thyroid hormone response. mRNA leaves the nucleus to make new proteins that encourage the function of the thyroid hormones, therefore increasing metabolic rate.

Increasing the metabolic rate can have various positive effects, depending on the target cell. It can:

- Aid in the development of brain cells

- Help skeletal and muscular cells grow

- Increase basal metabolic rate

- Improve circulation

**The Thyroid Gland: Conclusion**

Thyroid hormones are not easy to make; the process is very complicated and a lot could go wrong in the middle of the process. This makes probing for problems a lot harder because you cannot just look at the end product and come up with an accurate prognosis; you have to somehow think of various ways as to how the process could have gone wrong somewhere.

The thyroid gland is not it's own boss; it takes orders from the pituitary gland so that it knows how much T3 and T4 to make. In an ideal world, the pituitary gland always gives the right orders while the thyroid gland always follows those orders. Unfortunately, we live in a chaotic world where ideals break. In the next chapter you'll learn just how wonderfully complex your body is and just how important your thyroid gland is.

# Chapter 2: The Body as an Intelligent Machine

As a quick recap, the thyroid gland is that butterfly-shaped gland located in front of your neck just below your Adam's apple. While this gland may seemingly play an unimportant role compared to the heart or the brain, your body can't function properly without it.

You've probably heard of the word metabolism a couple of times in your life. People said to have quick metabolisms are often slender while people said to have slow metabolisms are often overweight. In a nutshell, people with fast metabolisms burn energy fast as well whereas people with slow metabolisms burn energy slow. The thyroid gland plays a vital role in your body as it controls your body's metabolism. A molecule called adenosine triphosphate (ATP) is what gives you energy. In order to make ATP, your body has to convert the glucose from the food you eat through a very complex chain of chemical processes, all of which need the help of your thyroid gland.

## The Synergy of the Systems of your Body

The human body is wonderfully complex. Every system works hard to keep the body in a stable state. Energy is a wonderful, intangible currency that every person can't get enough of. In order for the body to have enough energy, it needs all of the necessary components working in an optimal state.

In the context of the thyroid gland, the thyroid gland produces thyroid hormones that cause various changes in cells to convert glucose to ATP. When you have enough ATP in your body, you have more energy to spend. When energy is spent, your body generates heat, which also keeps you warm and toasty. This is why healthy people are associated with a "warm, healthy glow".

Without adequate amounts of ATP, your body will still work, but you may not have much energy to spare. Lack of ATP in the context of the thyroid gland does not spring from the lack of nutrients, but often from an insufficient amount of thyroid hormones that help convert glucose to ATP. Imagine eating a full meal packed with vitamins and minerals, only to feel half-full.

Just as nobody can survive without energy, nobody can survive without a thyroid gland. While a damaged thyroid may not have as quick of an effect as a heart attack, it's a guaranteed slow and painful death unless corrective steps are taken. If your thyroid completely ceases to work, you'd probably have one year left to live unless you get thyroid replacement therapy.

## Hormones: A Delicate Balance to be Maintained

The thyroid hormones stimulate the mitochondria to produce energy. Logically, there has to be enough thyroid hormones for the mitochondria to be able to produce plenty of energy. When your thyroid gland produces enough thyroid hormones and the cells in your body are able to use them properly, the result is an abundance of energy with all of the systems in your body performing at their best. Your brain can easily make decisions, remember things, and organize thoughts pretty fast. Your immune system is ready to fight virtually any disease.

You could easily lose or gain weight depending on what's appropriate. You have a feeling of alertness, enthusiasm, and joy knowing that you can juggle your daily tasks efficiently with energy left to spare. Then the excess energy produced by the cells turns to heat and provides you with that warm comfort commonly associated with intimate and happy memories.

In order to have a normal metabolism, there has to be a healthy amount of thyroid hormones produced and they also have to be used properly by the cells as well. Thyroid hormones not only affect your level of energy, immunity, and weight, but they also affect how your sugar levels, bone growth, muscle growth, heart rate, digestion, sleep, and more. This is because all of the systems in your body need energy to operate. Even in your sleep, your body keeps working. The most energy-hungry organ in your body is the brain. Consequently, it's the one that benefits the most from the energy produced by your thyroid glands.

### The Body as an Intelligent Machine - Conclusion

**The body truly is an intelligent machine; its complexity beats any modern human invention and until now its full potential has not yet been discovered. The thyroid gland is a silent worker, making sure that all of the other systems get enough fuel to perform at their best. The thyroid gland doesn't stand alone in this job though; it reports to the hypothalamus and the pituitary gland for specific instructions. You've seen that the process of synthesizing and distributing T3 and T4 is not a simple matter. The problem with such a high level of complexity is that plenty of things could easily go wrong; a simple error in gene production could lead to severe abnormalities. Even with the humongous chances of catastrophic failure due to the chaotic nature of the environment, the body fights on – an intelligent machine indeed.**

# Chapter 3: Thyroid Problems: Common Causes

Back in chapter 2, we've talked about how the systems of the body work together. While some organs may play a bigger role than others, they all need to function properly otherwise the body may not perform as expected. While the body is a very intelligent and efficient machine, it takes time to adapt and evolve when the environment changes. Our culture changes faster than our bodies can adapt to, which inevitably result to miscalculations and errors on our bodies' part. We commonly refer to them as diseases.

The thyroid gland helps your body produce the energy that various systems need, but what could possibly go wrong with this setup? Simplifying things, we could say that if the thyroid hormones are not created properly, are not created in sufficient numbers, or are not being used properly, then it's safe to say that symptoms of disease will inevitably pop up soon. When the small but important thyroid fails to do its job properly, which is to regulate the body's metabolism, several problems can occur. Here are some of the most common diseases usually associated with a malfunctioning thyroid gland:

- Hashimoto's Disease
- Graves' Disease
- Goiter
- Thyroid Nodules

Unfortunately a lot of thyroid problems go unnoticed because a lot of tests used in checking the thyroid function can only detect a small number of diseases. As mentioned in the previous chapters, the body's systems are interconnected – problems with the thyroid could come from other malfunctioning systems of the body. Problems with the thyroid may be tricky to find, so here's a few components that directly affect your thyroid:

- Thyroid Releasing Hormone (TRH)
- Thyroid Stimulating Hormone (TSH)
- Thyroxine (T4)
- Triiodothyronine (T3)
- Reverse T3 (RT3)
- Thyroid Antibodies

The roles played by these components shall be discussed in the succeeding chapters. Let's first go through the most common thyroid gland problems:

Hashimoto's disease: This is one of the leading causes of hypothyroidism. When your immune system attacks the thyroid gland like it's some kind of invader, then it can't do it's job properly and may eventually stop working altogether. Symptoms are pretty generic and could easily be attributed to old age. Fatigue, constipation, and depression are just some of the symptoms. In order to test for this disorder, doctors check the levels of TSH compared to the levels of thyroid hormone. If TSH is high but T3 and T4 are low, the test returns positive. Abnormal antibodies that attack the thyroid are also pretty obvious signs.

Graves' Disease: This is actually the most common cause of hyperthyroidism. The immune system also attacks the thyroid gland, but instead of producing less thyroid hormone, it produces a lot more. Because the thyroid gland produces so much T3 and T4, the body's metabolism speeds up to a dangerous rate. People with Graves' disease often find it hard to sleep and are also prone to panic attacks. Blood tests comparing the levels of TSH and T4 will see whether the patient has Graves' disease or not. Patients who have a huge amount of T4 and low levels of TSH are thought to have Graves' disease.

Goiter: The thyroid gland is enlarged. This is usually due to iodine deficiency. Another common cause is hyperthyroidism. In its starting phase, patients reported feeling of tightness in the neck, breathing or swallowing problems, coughing, and more. In most cases though, the proof is the enlarged goiter that's pretty visible anyway.

Thyroid Nodules: They are unwelcome growths that form on or inside the thyroid gland. A lot of these are harmless, but some can be cancerous.

## Chapter 3: Thyroid Problems: Common Causes: Conclusion

The thyroid gland doesn't just conk out on its own; miscommunication with the other systems of the body could cause this hardworking gland to make a lot of mistakes. The contrast of the thyroid hormones and TSH is often very important because it could pinpoint which organ, tissue, or cell is misbehaving.

The body sends out these complicated messages to help use pinpoint the possible roots of whatever is keeping the body from achieving a state of harmony. It's best to listen to it and hear what it has to say. In the next chapter we'll talk about how the body talks to you through various types of symptoms and diseases.

# Chapter 4: Thyroid Problems: Signs and Symptoms

Thyroid problems often go misdiagnosed because their symptoms are so common. A lot of doctors dismiss them as normal signs of aging instead of being real symptoms of an underlying problem with the thyroid gland. One of the most commonly misdiagnosed problems with the thyroid gland is hypothyroidism. If you've experienced fatigue, unexplained weight gain, insomnia, anxiety, depression, forgetfulness, severely lowered sex drive, infections that just won't go away, accelerated aging, among other symptoms, then you may be in fact, a hypothyroid sufferer.

Hypothyroidism is a slow disease. It just appears on your doorstep, slowly invading your body. Usually one or two symptoms appear and then as years go by, the rest of the symptoms manifest themselves so slowly that you'd think that your body is degrading due to the natural effects of aging. A lot of patients who experience these symptoms consult their doctors only to be told that what they're experiencing is normal while prescribing a bunch of synthetic drugs full of side effects.

In this chapter, you'll find useful information in finding out if you have hypothyroidism and the adverse effects it could have in your life. If you find that you have a lot of the symptoms mentioned in this chapter, consider seeking treatment as soon as possible. This chapter also aims to make you more vigilant and inquisitive especially regarding health issues.

### How do I Know if my Thyroid has a Problem?

In general, if your thyroid has a problem you'd usually have muscle and joint pain, carpal tunnel syndrome, hair loss and brittleness, dry skin, constipation, diarrhea, swelling neck, irregular periods, and more. As you see, the symptoms are pretty common and could easily be mistaken for other diseases or simply bad lifestyle choices.

### How do I Know if I have Hypothyroidism?

Fatigue and obesity are not the only symptoms of hypothyroidism. As we have already discussed in Chapter 2, the body is a wonderfully complex and intelligent machine; it will have different ways to tell you when something goes wrong. Because all the systems in your body require energy to work, a decrease in energy production may cause headaches, depression, digestive problems, cognitive dissonance, infertility, and more. Here are some of the symptoms that often occur to patients with hypothyroidism:

- Uncontrollable weight gain

- Relatively cold body, mostly on the hands and feet

- Impaired mental focus

- Fatigue

- Insomnia or low quality sleep

- Numbness or tingling in extremities

- Enlarged thyroid gland

- Brittle nails

- Mood swings

- Joint and muscle pain

- Constipation

- Headaches

- Prone to infections

- Irregular periods

- Infertility

- Miscarriage

- Decrease in sex drive

- Hypertension

- Dry skin

- Decreased sweating

- Pale complexion

- Hyper allergies

- Slowness in thinking (especially when talking)

- Fluid retention

Of course, you don't have to have all of these symptoms to have hypothyroidism. Every person will have different symptoms for hypothyroidism. If you've experienced some of these symptoms, then you may be hypothyroid.

**The Problem with Conventional Hypothyroid Tests**

A lot of doctors often rely on blood tests and other more quantifiable tests in order to diagnose patients. A lot of times though patients tell the doctors all they need to know. Lab tests should not be the only sole source of information used in diagnosing people.

It's important not only to check the blood of the patient, but also the medical history and the symptoms mentioned by the patient as well. Physical exams should also be done to probe for other physical manifestations of hypothyroidism.

Low body temperature is a common symptom of hypothyroidism, so if your temperature falls below the healthy body temperature, which is 98.6, then it implies that your body has a low metabolism, which may be caused by hypothyroidism.

The problem is that even if you manifest some of the symptoms of a low thyroid, if the blood tests come back normal, which means that your thyroid stimulating hormone (TSH) level is normal, they'd cross hypothyroidism out of the list immediately.

As mentioned back in chapter 1, the thyroid gland doesn't make the TSH; the pituitary gland does. The assumption made here is that if the pituitary gland makes enough TSH, most likely the thyroid gland makes enough T3 and T4.

**Temperature as a Thyroid Health Monitor**

Because your body produces heat when excess energy is made, your pituitary gland will monitor your body's temperature and tell your thyroid gland to produce the appropriate amount of hormones depending on how hot your body needs to be. If it's too cold, your pituitary gland will make more TSH so that the thyroid gland will make more T3 and T4. Otherwise, it'll tell your thyroid gland to lower the production of T3 and T4.

If you feel cold or hot when others don't, you may want to check if you have other symptoms of hypothyroidism. Some of the symptoms are quite subtle, so be observant. Even if you're told that there is nothing wrong with you based on lab tests, trust your instincts. If it doesn't feel right, it probably isn't. Oftentimes when you manifest symptoms of hypothyroidism without being flagged as having a low thyroid, it's often your pituitary gland that's conking out and needs to be fixed.

**Aging and Its Effects on Hormone Production**

Aging presents a world of complications for the unsuspecting adult. Cancer, stroke, arthritis, and a lot more diseases seem to pop out of nowhere. The body seems to be more prone to disease as it gets older. Like most machines, your body will eventually wear down, especially since a lot of important hormones start to decrease in production. The three hormones: thyroid hormones, sex hormones, and adrenal hormones get a steady decrease in production. This is perhaps why a lot of doctors dismiss symptoms of hypothyroidism as a simple effect of aging.

Here are a few other factors other than aging that lead to the decline of thyroid hormones production:

- Treatment from hyperthyroidism

- Medications that inhibit the cells in your body to use T3 and T4 properly

- Autoimmune disease

- Infections

## Obesity as an Indicator of a Low Functioning Thyroid

Obesity is one of the most common symptoms of a low functioning thyroid because a lot of people with hypothyroidism tend to have very low metabolism. It was mentioned before that a lower than normal body temperature is an almost sure sign of hypothyroidism. This has to do with the connection of body temperature and metabolism.

Your body's metabolism is affected not just by the thyroid hormones; it is affected by a lot of biochemical reactions that happen all around your body. The thyroid hormones triiodothyronine (T3) and thyroxine (T4) are vital components for a normal metabolism though. Recall from chapter 1 that T3 is about ten times more active than T4. This means that T4 has to be converted so that the cells can use it to make ATP, which as you may recall, is the energy currency of the body. There is no workaround; the cells will only accept T3. While this may seem easy, your body could convert T4 into another thyroid hormone called reverse T3 (RT3). This type of thyroid hormone blocks T3 receptor sites effectively preventing cells from using it. Ideally, there aren't enough RT3 in your system to cause much problems, but when that delicate balance is broken, problems will inevitably arise.

## Stress and Hypothyroidism

Stress is one of the root causes of a lot of system failures in the body. In the past, stress is used by the body as a defense mechanism; your heart rate is elevated, you become more alert, and pretty much your survival instincts kick into high gear. This happens to ensure that you can escape predators and live to spread your genes. However, as intricate and complex as your body many be, it still hasn't caught up in modern society. In the past, people only experienced stress in short bursts. Now people experience them in dangerously extended periods of time, often reaching even a couple of years!

Whether you experience short-term stress or long-term stress, the chemical released is the same: cortisol. Cortisol is sent out by the body to deal with stress. When this chemical is released, your body changes its state from a restful, healing one to an alert, aggressive one. This is the reason why you feel like you have superpowers when you're about to reach a deadline. The body has its limits though and if you stay in a cortisol-fueled state, your body becomes prone to disease. You see, in order for the body to boost other functions like alertness and strength, it has to decrease other functions like immunity to disease.

Another problem with cortisol is that it prevents the conversion of T4 to T3. Instead, it encourages the conversion of T4 to RT3. When you look at it from an evolutionary perspective, it doesn't seem to make sense because why would you want to reduce ATP production when the body really needs energy in stressful moments? Then again, the body is complex and it might not have needed to prevent this mechanism from happening in the past.

## Allergies and Hypothyroidism

Allergies happen when your immune system thinks of something harmless as an invader and continually tries to get rid of it. This uses up energy and causes a lot of trouble, especially when swelling happens near blood vessels and air pathways. Hypothyroidism is thought to cause chronic allergies. This does make sense considering that a compromised immune system is more likely to make wrong predictions and decisions as compared to a perfectly functional immune system. Hypothyroidism causes ATP to be produced in much lesser numbers, hence potentially causing a decline in the immune response.

People with allergies often have to buy antihistamines to suppress the immune system false alarms otherwise they experience these symptoms:

- Difficulty breathing
- Fatigue
- Colds
- Headaches
- Coughs
- Skin rashes
- Gastrointestinal problems
- Swelling

If these symptoms happen to you at rather predictable times, you may have allergies. Antihistamines are quick fixes that don't really help you get better in the long run. Instead, opt for allergy treatment to slowly acclimate your immune system to the false positives so that your immune system won't overreact to harmless pollens floating around in spring.

If you want to know what you're allergic to, skin tests are often pretty accurate. When you get the list of things you're allergic to, get allergy drops so you can begin desensitizing yourself to various allergens on your list.

**Thyroid Self-Checks**

Here's how to do a quick thyroid neck check:

1. Stand in front of a mirror close enough so you can see your neck where the thyroid gland is located

2. Tip your head back

3. Swallow

4. Look out for any anomalies as you swallow

Repeat this many times in order to get more accurate results. If you see anomalies when you swallow, consult a doctor immediately.

Another way to check if your thyroid hormones aren't doing their job is to put a thermometer in your mouth and measure your temperature. If your temperature falls 1-2 degrees below 98.6 degrees, chances are you have hypothyroidism especially if you experience fatigue quite a lot.

**Chapter 4: Thyroid Problems: Signs and Symptoms: Conclusion**

While blood tests may be able to provide quantitative results, which are often pretty accurate, the interpretation of results come from clinical trials and research on animals and humans. This leaves plenty of room for improvement as well as error. The problem with blood tests is that a lot of the information they contain is from the body's present state. Thyroid diseases often have cumulative effects that could scatter symptoms over different timelines.

The body could also send out different signs and symptoms based on the organs that need repair. If multiple organs need repair, oftentimes the signs and symptoms become a lot more difficult to decode. Hypothyroidism remains one of the most misdiagnosed diseases because the symptoms are similar to a lot of diseases. Then it was found out that some diseases with similar symptoms might have actually caused each other.

The threshold for normal TSH is also biased in terms of age. Older people are expected to have anomalies in the thyroid hormone production of their bodies. This is why a lot of doctors dismiss symptoms of a malfunctioning thyroid as mere effects of aging.

If you suspect that you may have thyroid problems based on the symptoms and self-checks you've just read, don't hesitate to ask your doctor about it. The earlier you get yourself diagnosed, the better.

# Chapter 5: Hypertension and Hypothyroidism: The Interconnection

Given that a lot of symptoms of hypothyroidism are also manifested by other diseases, it's a logical assumption that whatever is causing trouble with thyroid hormone production or utilization could also be causing trouble with other systems of the body. Another valid assumption is that one disease causes another. The body needs all the systems to cooperate, and if one system fails to do its job properly, other systems won't be able to perform at their best.

## The Heart and the Thyroid

Heart ailments are becoming increasingly common due to the unhealthy lifestyle that prevails in most societies. The heart is tasked with pumping blood to all of the systems that need it. When a system has trouble receiving the blood pumped by the heart, the heart works harder to deliver the same amount of blood. When a system fails to receive the blood pumped by the heart, other systems may also suffer due to blood vessels possibly bursting or blood not going to them as well.

With such a large duty entrusted unto the thyroid, it's no surprise that problems with the thyroid would mean problems with the heart as well. That being said, one of the prevailing yet unsuspected causes of heart ailments is hypothyroidism.

While correlation does not equal causation, it was speculated that people who had strong and well functioning thyroids had lesser chances of having heart ailments. The hypothesis does make sense, as the thyroid gland is in charge of creating ATP that is the energy currency of the body. When the thyroid gland fails to produce the much needed T3 and T4, the body as a whole weakens, the heart along with it.

## The Immune System and the Thyroid

Some medical experts who have explored several options in strengthening the immune system of their patients have tried giving their patients desiccated thyroid hormone supplements. The immune system of the patients grew stronger, being able to fight a lot of diseases than before. They found out that the patients with the most significant improvements are the ones who had hypothyroidism. They then concluded that the thyroid plays a huge role in keeping your body free of diseases. This is why a lot of people catch more diseases as they age; the amount of thyroid hormones in their bodies are much lower.

## Hypertension and Hypothyroidism

Because the heart and the thyroid both need to perform at their best, if one of them breaks down, the other one breaks down as well. A lot of doctors are currently looking into the correlation of hypertension and hypothyroidism because a lot of patients come with both ailments instead of just one. Hypothyroidism is said to impair the heart's ability to pump blood, therefore possibly leading to a heart attack. Furthermore, people who've taken steps to improve the thyroid hormone production in their body were shown to have decreased occurrences of angina and a much lower chance of heart failure.

The connection found between hypothyroidism and hypertension is quite revolutionary. Synthetic drugs prescribed for hypertension only alleviates the pain but it doesn't actually fix the problem. These synthetic drugs also have a lot of side effects that severely decrease the quality of life of the people who take them. The worst part is that once you're given medication for hypertension, you cannot stop taking it anymore.

One of the realizations that led to the discovery of a connection between hypothyroidism and hypertension was that patients who were treated for hypothyroidism suddenly showed signs of improvements in their overall health, effectively removing hypertension medication from their lives. Whether the patients had naturally healthy lifestyles or dangerously neglected lifestyles, the results were the same; their hearts sprang back to life, alleviating a lot of symptoms brought about by both hypertension and hypothyroidism.

## The War Against Cholesterol

A lot of people talk about cholesterol as if it's an ominous entity bent on destroying their bodies. If this is the case then that means our bodies are always set on self-destruct mode as every cell we have is ready to make cholesterol should our bodies require it.

Ever since heart attacks were associated with high levels of cholesterol, people have begun seeing it as an enemy. A lot of clinical trials regarding the dangers of cholesterol were done on animals, some of which cannot use cholesterol at all, leading to the overall degradation of their bodies and eventual death. Unrealistically huge amounts of cholesterol were also given in a controlled environment. As you may already know, too much of anything will almost always cause harm. Unfortunately, test results from clinical trials are almost always sensationalized by the media. Pretty soon false data starts to spread like poison, leading to false assumptions and claims about the effects of cholesterol in the body.

Because of this "breakthrough" wherein people thought they've discovered the culprit in hypertension, more rushed studies were done in order to prove the findings regarding the bad effects of cholesterol on the body. Heart ailments were rashly correlated to low cholesterol diets.

Strangely, a lot of heart ailments are not exactly caused by cholesterol. The body responds to different types of stimuli and will send signals depending on what it experiences. Usually when the levels of cholesterol in the body increase, it means that the body is trying to heal injured parts, which in the heart's case are the arteries. A lot of studies link heart ailments to high cholesterol when only a correlation is found. This means that high cholesterol levels doesn't necessarily cause heart ailments – it's just commonly found in people with heart ailments.

**Two Birds with One Stone**

In order to prevent or control hypertension, people have been trying to lower their cholesterol levels even if they fall within the normal range. While this method may alleviate some of the symptoms of hypertension, it's a rather shortsighted approach that leads to a lifetime of expensive medications with side effects.

Just as proper thyroid hormone production and usage leads to proper functioning of the body's systems, inadequate thyroid hormone supply and usage will inevitably lead to various types of diseases, hypertension being one of them. What exactly binds hypertension and hypothyroidism though? Are they both caused by a certain deficiency or damage? A prime suspect lies in the citadel that protects you from foreign invaders. Patients with hypothyroidism are found to have huge amounts of mucin accumulating in the tissues in an abnormal manner, therefore causing swelling. Unlike cholesterol that the body uses as a building block, mucin is found to be a direct cause of the swelling that spreads to all of the connective tissues in your body. It causes a lot of symptoms commonly associated with hypothyroidism such as water retention and swelling.

Because the heart has a lot of connective tissues, huge amounts of mucin could potentially damage the delicate components like the arteries. Eventually this leads to erratic pumping of blood. When your heart no longer pumps blood efficiently, it changes. It finds other ways to get blood into your other systems, causing it to work a lot harder than it needs to and therefore severely reducing its lifespan.

When hypertension medications are used, oftentimes the source of the problem is not addressed. Instead, the symptoms are covered and the real root of the problem becomes harder to find. Some medications cause vasodilation, which increases the size of the blood vessels and therefore making more room for blood to flow. Some medications cause the heart to pump slower, therefore effectively reducing the blood pressure but also inevitably causing tiredness and fatigue due to inadequate amounts of blood circulating the system. These medications are also temporary; your body won't learn how to do the things they do, so you'll have to take them regularly just to have a normal life.

A lot of times the solution to a problem isn't straightforward; you can't look for a solution just based on the present state. In the context of hypertension, you can't just patch up problems as they come along; you have to remember that systems of the body work together, and if one part malfunctions, the others most likely will malfunction as well. Hypertension may just be an indicator of a low functioning thyroid and could therefore be remedied by taking natural thyroid supplements. In fact, some patients who have started to take natural thyroid supplements show immediate signs of improvement, such as the shrinking of the enlarged heart back to its normal size and more importantly, the alleviation of hypertension. The amount of mucin present also decreases.

## Chapter 5: Hypertension and Hypothyroidism: The Interconnection: Conclusion

One of the most common disease that severely decreases the quality of life is more preventable and curable than you think. Hypertension and hypothyroidism share a lot of symptoms and are suspected to be connected by this key component called mucin. A lot of research and results from clinical trials have been sensationalized to put cholesterol in bad light. Hypothyroidism is commonly associated with high cholesterol levels, but another important fact that a lot of people miss is that it's also associated with high levels of mucin. Cholesterol is essential in keeping a healthy and fit body, therefore using synthetic drugs to lower them may not actually cure hypertension; it might just hide it. On the other hand, natural thyroid hormone supplements were shown to actually lower the amount of mucin present in the body, therefore reducing swelling and effectively helping the body achieve a state of stability again. When that happens, it can enter a state of healing and further lower the risk of any fatal disease.

It's particularly tricky to diagnose one of the most complex machineries ever created - the human body. It's pretty easy to just patch up holes and hope for the best, but in the long run those patches will give way. The best way to heal your body is to listen to it. If you have overlapping symptoms of hypothyroidism and hypertension, you may opt to try natural thyroid hormone supplementation. The earlier you start healing your thyroid the faster your body can go back to its happy, perky state.

# Chapter 6: Problems with Conventional Medicine

The usual suggested solutions in western medicine are:

- Surgery
- Hormone replacement drugs
- Radiation
- Various Pharmaceutical Drugs

Levothyroxine is usually suggested and recommended by the FDA. While it's enough to make a patient "survive", it often brings along a bunch of side effects including nausea, vomiting, diarrhea, headaches, insomnia, increased appetite, weight loss, heat sensitivity, hair loss, angina, irregular heartbeat, and more. Ironically a lot of these side effects are also symptoms of hypothyroidism.

Western medicine demystified a lot of concepts about thyroid hormones and what they do. The problem is that there are so many diseases that your intricately made and complex body could catch. Your body will give out different signs and symptoms to tell you what it's currently doing to fight diseases while also telling you what it needs you to do to fight it.

A lot of thyroid treatments bring more harm to your body than good because some doctors prefer to patch the symptoms one by one instead of finding the root cause of the symptoms and working on that instead. Imagine a patient who just has a few symptoms of hypothyroidism. The doctor then prescribes drugs to stop the symptoms, only to have a few more pop up due to side effects. Eventually this patient goes to another doctor, who then misdiagnoses the patient due to the misleading symptoms. This goes on and on until the patient has a bunch of expensive medications with a plethora of side effects and still no relief.

It's important to know what happens inside your body so that you can protect yourself from harmful medications and you can describe your situation to the doctors better for more accurate and safe medications.

## Chapter 6: Problems with Conventional Medicine: Conclusion

Western medicine presents a great leap in human health, but it still stumbles every now and then. While a lot of medicines offer a quick fix to plenty of diseases, they are merely patches that could make the problems worsen over time. Western medicine relies strongly on results of various clinical trials and researches, but sometimes it fails to take into account a more humane approach in dealing with disease. It can delve too much into the numbers, forgetting that patients are also human.

Just because your doctor makes mistakes doesn't mean you have to stop following everything he says; it just means you have to be more vigilant and aware on what happens inside your body.

# Chapter 9: Natural Cures

As mentioned in the previous chapters, there is a powerful interconnection of the systems of the body. The complex interaction between these systems require adequate amounts of vitamins and minerals to work properly. With an abundant source of vitamins and minerals, the body can build and repair itself while being able to fight off foreign invaders. The thyroid gland is one of the organs that benefit strongly from the addition of vitamins and minerals (assuming that the ones taking them are vitamin-and-mineral-deficient ). Here are some of the vitamins and minerals that you could benefit from if you're suffering from a low functioning thyroid:

High-quality multivitamins: While it is possible to live a life free from supplements, it requires a steady supply of organic food, which would be quite expensive to maintain. If you live in an urban city, chances are a lot of the foods you eat contain significantly less vitamins and minerals than the foods found in rural cities. High quality multivitamins help you get the vitamins and minerals you may have missed from your diet.

A lot of cheap multivitamins may look like they have plenty of vitamins and minerals because of the above-100% daily recommended dosage, but truth it's often just a marketing ploy. The problem with cheap multivitamins is that they use non-chelated minerals, which are less bioavailable than chelated minerals. This means that they are harder to absorb by the body and therefore only part of the vitamins and minerals are used. High-quality multivitamins use chelated minerals, which are more bioavailable and therefore could easily be absorbed by the body. This is why cheap multivitamins have to increase the amount of vitamins and minerals present in order to compensate for its low bioavailability. The problem here is that the more synthetic vitamins and minerals consume the harder your kidney needs to work. High quality multivitamins have the right amount of nutrients your body need without overworking your kidney.

A good indicator that the multivitamin you're buying is high quality is that it uses the bioavailable methylcobalamin for vitamin B12 instead of its less bioavailable counterpart, cyanocobalamin. A lot of cheap multivitamins particularly like switching substituting methylcobalamin for cyanocobalamin to cut costs. Invest in high quality multivitamins that does not cut corners so you get the full health benefits like a boosted immune system, a healthy circulation, and of course a healthy thyroid gland.

Fish oil: Fish oil is hailed often as a magic bullet in the brain, usually boosting the ability of the brain to memorize and analyze data. You may opt for a diet rich in omega-3 fatty acids, but if you're in a situation wherein you still are deficient in omega-3 fatty acids, then you may want to buy fish oil. Oftentimes higher quality fish oil would mean less fishy aftertaste and smell, but in most cases it's safe to use cheap fish oil.

Fish oil is not only found to boost cognitive functions, but it's also found to improve thyroid hormone production.

Vitamin D: Vitamin D is one of the most common vitamins available, yet a lot of people are found to be deficient in it. People deficient in vitamin D are often more prone to getting heart ailments and other diseases. A lot of people with low functioning thyroids tend to have low levels of vitamin D, so you can either get more by spending more time outside or by taking vitamin D supplements. If you've already invested in high quality multivitamins, chances are vitamin D is already covered.

Vitamin D: Many hypothyroid patients have low levels of vitamin D. A deficiency in vitamin D increases your risk for major diseases such as cancer, heart disease, and osteoporosis. Have your physician check your 25-hydroxy vitamin D level and consider optimizing your vitamin D level.

Selenium: Antioxidants are always welcome in the body due to their cancer-fighting properties. Selenium not only helps get rid of free radicals that damage your system, but it also helps convert T4 to T3.

Iodine: One of the root causes of hypothyroidism is a constant shortage of iodine. While this is becoming less common due to the huge amount of salts present in most foods, a lot of people still have low levels of iodine in their system. A healthy thyroid gland is one with adequate amounts of iodine. If you have a low functioning thyroid due to iodine shortage, it only makes sense to add iodine in your diet in the form of iodized salt. Otherwise you may just take iodine supplements to help stimulate healthy thyroid hormone production.

L-Tyrosine: L-Tyrosine is an amino acid that helps the thyroid hormones do their jobs properly, therefore lack of L-Tyrosine would often cause symptoms similar to that of hypothyroidism. In fact, low amounts of L-Tyrosine in the body were often linked with a low functioning thyroid. Make sure that your body has enough L-Tyrosine.

## FOODS FOR A HEALTHIER THYROID

Eat less: Goitrogens are compounds that often prevent **retention** the thyroid from doing its job properly. It's found in a lot of vegetation and is more common than you might think. If you suffer from low thyroid function you may opt to eat less:

- Brussels sprouts

- Cabbage

- Turnips

- Rutabaga

- Radishes

- Cauliflower

- Broccoli

- Kale

- Soy millet

You may have heard of the gluten-free fad and perhaps even tried it yourself. A lot of people dismiss the gluten-free concept as a marketing ploy to get people to buy more expensive products out of the fear that they could have severe allergies to it. For people who have hypothyroidism, however, a gluten-free diet may not be such a bad idea. Here's why:

Hashimoto's thyroidism, which is a condition wherein the immune system makes a colossal mistake of attacking the thyroid tissue, is a common cause of hypothyroidism. Because the molecular structure and composition of the gluten protein and the human thyroid tissue look almost identical, the immune system may also start attacking gluten. The longer the immune system fights, the more energy it depletes. People with hypothyroidism already have severely decreased levels of energy, so if you have a low functioning thyroid you may want to avoid foods with gluten.

Eat more: It was mentioned earlier that you need certain nutrients like iodine in order for your thyroid gland to function properly. If you can find foods already rich in the nutrients aforementioned, it's best to consume that instead of buying supplements. Here are other foods known to have various nutrients that supercharges thyroid function:

Iodine-rich foods:

- Fish
- Meat
- Eggs
- Certain seafood
- Potatoes
- Navy beans
- Oats
- Himalayan salt
- Parsley

Tyrosine-rich food:

- Avocados
- Bananas
- Pumpkin seeds
- Lentils

- Almonds

Bladderwrack gets a special mention, as it's a seaweed plant jam-packed with nutrients. It contains a lot of iodine, potassium, calcium, zinc, and more vitamins and minerals. Also, it's been thought that this type of seaweed actually stimulates the thyroid gland.

Coconut oil is also shown to promote metabolism just as thyroid hormones do. When combined, they form a powerful synergy. Two tablespoons of extra virgin coconut oil daily should be enough to yield noticeable results. You may swallow the oil directly or combine it with other food.

Healthy fats are important components in building hormonal pathways. By consuming foods rich in healthy fats, you can help your body rebuild and repair itself. Here are some of the foods rich in healthy fats:

- Avocados
- Nuts
- Dairy products
- Meat and fish
- Flax seeds
- Coconut oil
- Fish oil

### The Immune System and the Stomach

The digestive system and the immune system are said to be highly related. It's even said that Hashimoto's thyroiditis and other thyroid problems spring from damage from the digestive system. Drinking a probiotic drink everyday is said to be able to help your digestive system withstand more stomach health problems.

### Yoga

Because stress is often the main cause of a lot of diseases, it's only natural that exercises that alleviate stress also alleviate these diseases. Consistent yoga sessions can actually help you alleviate the symptoms of various ailments, especially thyroid problems. A lot of chronic ailments are said to easily be relieved due to the balance and harmony created inside the body.

### Chapter 9: Natural Cures: Conclusion

Synthetic drugs are often made to 'fix' a disease as quickly as it can. When you take synthetic drugs, you confuse the body by making it think that the substances its using came from its own system, therefore it trusts the medication and lets it do often whatever it wants. The guard is now down and if the medication suddenly wrecks havoc in some other system in order to fulfill its duty, the body has to pay the consequences. Side effects are often pretty good reasons not to use synthetic drugs. A lot of short-term side effects are pretty unbearable. A lot of clinical trials have not tested modern drugs for their long-term side effects, hence, synthetic drugs may have negative long term side-effects yet to be seen. Natural cures and remedies on the other hand, have been tested by nature itself for millions of years. Plants and animals have evolved alongside humans, adapting to the quickly changing environment.

Surprisingly a lot of foods that can help you get your thyroid gland back into shape are actually pretty common. Unfortunately the foods you should be avoiding are also quite common. Be mindful of the foods you eat so that you won't have to get stuck into a vortex of eternal medication.

Exercise plays a huge role in keeping your thyroid healthy because it helps alleviate stress. Stress is a dangerous thyroid destroyer, so avoid prolonged stress.

In a nutshell, the best way to nurse your thyroid back to perfect health is to remove prolonged stress from your life. Healthful food and daily exercise can only do so much to help your body cope with the stress it's experiencing but if the stress overwhelms it, it sort of self-destructs; various organs start to fail and the body stops responding to medication. Nature has provided great ways to remove stress, so eat natural foods, exercise, and meditate

Lastly, remember that while a lot of these lifestyle changes and tweaks may improve thyroid function drastically, it's always important to keep in touch with your doctor. There have been incidences wherein people started self-medicating out of distrust and eventually caused irreversible damages on their own bodies. We live in a world with a lot of artificial creations. If severe damage to the thyroid gland is done by something man made, in most cases the cure is also man made. Natural remedies may not be able to alleviate the symptoms of a disease created by man. If the disease is still in its early stages though, natural remedies most likely could handle it.

# Conclusion

The body is a pretty powerful and complex machine. It has intricately-made systems that interact using a series of complex biochemical reactions. Proper communication of these systems is needed to maintain a strong and healthy body. As discussed in the previous chapters, problems with a certain system could easily cascade into various problems with other systems because of miscommunication - imagine being really sick and trying to relay important information to another person while running.

Hypothyroidism is one of the most common diseases of the thyroid but also one of the most misdiagnosed. It's often the cause of a lot of fatal diseases that severely decrease the quality of life of people unfortunate enough to catch it. Unfortunately, a lot of people do catch this disease especially when they grow older.

A lot of patients are misdiagnosed because of the exaggeration of the negative effects of getting old. Researchers often assume the worst as people age, therefore skewing the expected results of various research to check for hypothyroidism and other problems with the thyroid. With this as a major roadblock, patients often have to look for other ways to address their discomforts. Unfortunately, a lot of these other ways include unfounded "quack" medicine that could potentially make things a lot worse. On the other hand, prescription drugs often only patch the problem instead of really fixing it. Either way the patient seems to always be on the losing end.

Fortunately there is a way out. As shown in the previous chapters, your body is well equipped and can heal and defend itself if you allow it. Using natural cures and remedies with a bit of help from western medicine, you can have your life back in just a few days. Imagine having the vitality of your prime years back and being able to spend more time with your family while having extra energy to work and play. If you can have your life back by making a few lifestyle changes and tweaks, would you do it?

This book was written so that you can choose to turn your life around and live a healthy lifestyle. Natural thyroid supplementation with proper foods, exercise, vitamins, and minerals will help you get your health back in just a few days so you could make the best comeback you could ever imagine.

Thank you again for downloading this book!

I hope you enjoyed reading about my book on Nature's Remedy for Thyroid

Finally, if you enjoyed this book, please take the time to share your thoughts and **post a review on Amazon**.  It'd be greatly appreciated!

Thank you!

## Next Steps

- Write me an honest review about the book – I truly value your opinion and thoughts and I will incorporate them into my next book, which is already underway.

http://www.amazon.com/dp/B00LT1B1HU

www.ingramcontent.com/pod-product-compliance
Lightning Source LLC
Chambersburg PA
CBHW081807280526
45789CB00008B/3038